The Alkaline

Diet for Beginners

Delicious Alkaline Recipes to Lose Weight and Increase your Energy

Sam Carter

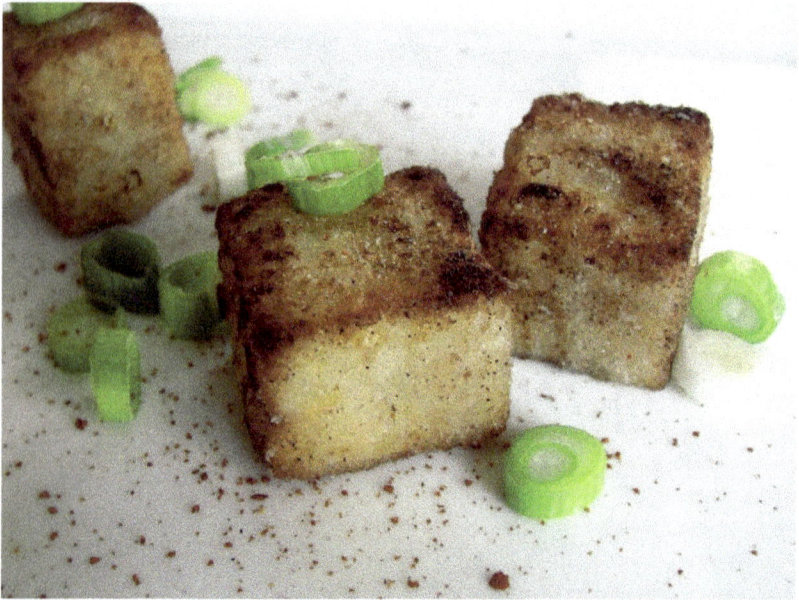

Please consult a licensed professional before attempting any techniques outlined in this book.

By reading this document, the reader agrees that under no circumstances is the author responsible for any losses, direct or indirect, which are incurred as a result of the use of information contained within this document, including, but not limited to, — errors, omissions, or inaccuracies.

Table of Contents

Autumn Salad

Servings: 2

Total Time: 35 minutes

Ingredients

- 1 large sweet potato, diced
- 2 beets, peeled and diced
- 2 tablespoons coconut oil
- ¼ teaspoon Himalayan salt
- 1 teaspoon black pepper
- ¼ cup almonds, toasted and chopped
- ¼ cup raisins
- 1 cup spinach, chopped
- ½ cup quinoa, cooked
- ¼ cup parsley, chopped

Dressing

- 2 tablespoons raw apple cider vinegar
- 1 lime, juiced
- ¼ cup extra virgin olive oil
- 1 teaspoon Himalayan salt

Directions

1.   Preheat oven to 350°F/180°C.

2.   In a small bowl, whisk together the vinegar, lime juice, olive oil and salt. Set aside.

3.   Place diced sweet potato and beets in a small bowl and pour in the coconut oil and sprinkle with salt and pepper. Toss well to coat and then arrange on a baking tray that has been lined with parchment paper.

4.   Roast the potato and beet in the oven for 25 minutes or until tender.

5.   In a large bowl, combine the sweet potato, beet, almonds, raisins, spinach, quinoa and parsley. Pour Dressing on top and toss well to coat.

6.   Serve immediately.

Nutty Tacos

Servings: 2

Total Time: 10 minutes

Ingredients

- ½ cup walnuts

- ¼ cup slivered raw almonds, blanched

- ¼ cup sun-dried tomatoes, soaked, drained, and roughly chopped

- 2 tablespoons olive oil

- 1 teaspoon ground cumin

- 1 teaspoon ground coriander

- ⅛ teaspoon chili powder

- ⅛ teaspoon garlic powder

- ⅛ teaspoon onion powder

- ⅛ teaspoon smoked paprika

- 1 teaspoon coconut aminos

- 1 teaspoon tamari

- ⅛ teaspoon Himalayan salt

- ¼ cup red quinoa, cooked

- 4-6 romaine lettuce leaves

- 2 tablespoons nutritional yeast

- 1 tablespoon chopped flat-leaf cilantro

Directions

1. Place walnuts and almonds in a food processor and pulse until chopped. Add in the sun-dried tomatoes and pulse a few times until mixed with the walnuts and almonds and mixture is crumbly.

2. Add in the olive oil, cumin, coriander, chili, garlic, onion, paprika, coconut aminos, tamari and salt. Pulse a few more times until combined.

3. Place nut and tomato mixture in a bowl and stir in the quinoa.

4. Divide mixture up amongst the romaine leaves and top with nutritional yeast and cilantro before serving.

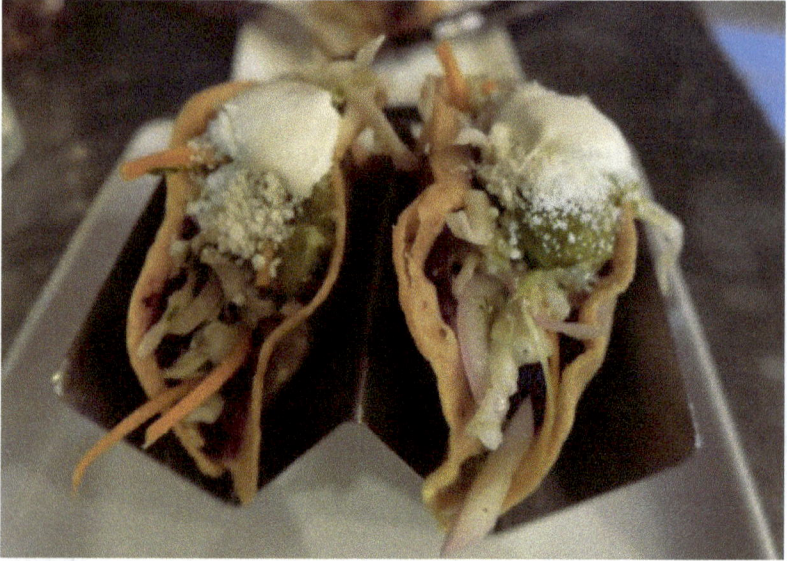

Cold Sesame Salad

Servings: 2

Total Time: 15 minutes

Ingredients

- 1 tablespoon avocado oil

- 1 large sweet potato, spiralized into noodles

- 1 large zucchini, spiralized into noodles

- 3 tablespoons tahini paste

- 1 ½ tablespoons toasted sesame oil

- 2 tablespoons raw apple cider vinegar

- 1 teaspoon raw honey

- 1 teaspoon lime juice

- 1 teaspoon coconut aminos

- 1 teaspoon tamari

- Pinch crushed red pepper flakes

- ⅛ teaspoon Himalayan salt

- 1 green onion, diced

- 1 tablespoon sesame seeds

Directions

1.   Heat avocado oil in a medium skillet over medium heat. Add sweet potato noodles and cooked 5 minutes, stirring occasionally. Add zucchini noodles and cook another 3 minutes before turning the heat to low.

2.   Whisk together the tahini, sesame oil, apple cider vinegar, honey, lime juice, coconut aminos, tamari and red pepper flakes in a small bowl.

3.   Pour tahini mixture over the noodles and toss to coat. Season with the salt and transfer to serving bowl.

4.   Let chill and then garnish with green onions and sesame seeds to serve.

Tex-Mex Bowl

Servings: 2

Total Time: 20 minutes plus 5 hours chill time

Ingredients

- 4 bell peppers, seeds and stems removed, sliced into strips
- 1 large red onion, thinly sliced
- 2 large garlic cloves, minced
- 2 oranges, juiced
- 1 lemon, zested and juiced
- 1 lime, zested and juiced
- ¼ cup apple cider vinegar
- ¼ cup olive oil
- ¼ teaspoon Himalayan salt
- 1 avocado, sliced
- 2 tablespoons cilantro
- 2 tablespoons nutritional yeast

Spiced Brown Rice

- 1 cup brown rice, cooked
- 2 teaspoons chili powder

- 1 ½ teaspoon garlic powder

- 1 teaspoon Himalayan salt

- 1 teaspoon paprika

- ½ teaspoon cayenne pepper

- ½ teaspoon garlic powder

- ½ cup black beans, drained and rinsed

Salsa

- 2 large tomatoes, diced

- ½ red onion, peeled and diced

- ¼ cup cilantro leaves, diced

- ¼ teaspoon salt

- juice of 1 lime

Directions

1. In a large bowl, combine the bell peppers, red onion, garlic, orange juice, lemon juice and zest, lime juice and zest, vinegar, olive oil and salt. Cover and let rest in the fridge for 5 hours.

2. While peppers marinate in the fridge, make the Salsa by combining all the Salsa ingredients in a small bowl. Stir well to combine, cover and place in the fridge.

3.   In a medium sized bowl, add together all the Spiced Brown Rice ingredients. Toss well and set aside.

4.   Heat a medium sized skillet over medium-high heat. Add bell peppers and a few tablespoons of the marinade. Sauté for 10 minutes or until the bell peppers and onions are soft.

5.   Place rice in serving bowls and top with bell pepper/onion mixture, sliced avocado, salsa and garnish with cilantro and nutritional yeast.

Stuffed Eggplant

Servings: 2

Total Time: 25 minutes

Ingredients

- 2 small eggplants, cut into ½ inch thin slices
- 2 tablespoons olive oil, divided
- 1 shallot, diced
- 1 teaspoon cumin
- ¼ teaspoon turmeric powder
- ¼ teaspoon cinnamon
- 1 tablespoon fresh ginger, grated
- ⅛ teaspoon cayenne pepper
- 1 large carrot, diced
- 1 cup quinoa, cooked
- 2 tablespoons raisins
- 1 tablespoon pine nuts, toasted
- 3 tablespoons parsley, chopped

Directions

1. Prepare eggplant by brushing with 1 tablespoon of the olive oil and placing on a grill pan or a baking tray. Broil in the oven on high for 4 minutes each side. Remove and set aside.

2. In a medium skillet over medium-low heat, add the shallot and cook for 3 minutes.

3. Add the cumin, turmeric, cinnamon, ginger and cayenne. Sauté for 1 minute before adding in the carrot. Continue cooking for another 8 minutes.

4. Transfer shallot and carrot mixture to a medium sized bowl and add the quinoa, raisins, pine nuts and parsley.

5. Place a small amount of the quinoa filling on each eggplant slice and roll up, securing with a toothpick before serving.

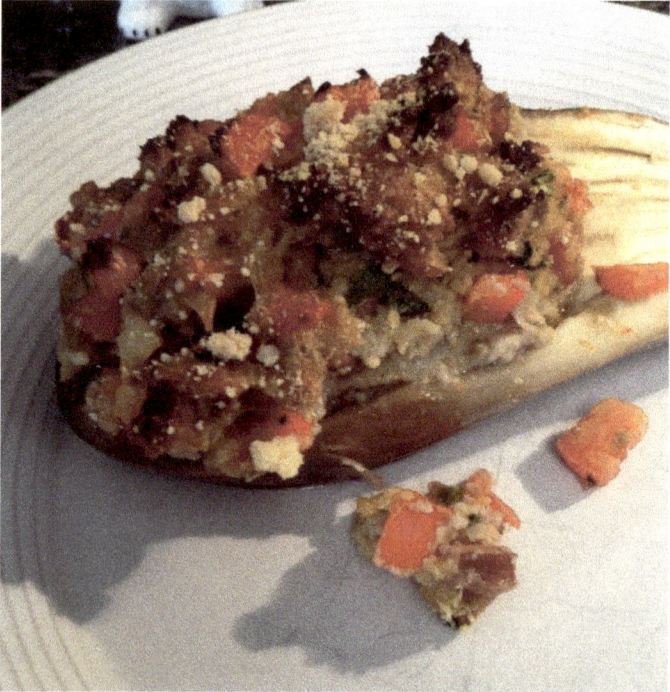

Chickpea Millet & Cucumber Salad

Servings: 2

Total Time: 10 minutes

Ingredients

- 1 garlic clove, minced
- 1 teaspoon cumin
- 1 teaspoon Himalayan salt
- 3 tablespoons avocado oil
- 2 tablespoons lemon juice
- 1 teaspoon lemon zest
- 1 teaspoon oregano
- 1 cup millet, cooked
- 1 cup cucumber, diced
- 1 cup chickpeas, drained + rinsed
- 3 cups spinach, chopped
- 2 tablespoons parsley, chopped
- 2 tablespoons black olives, chopped

Directions

1.   In a small bowl, whisk together the garlic, cumin, salt, avocado oil, lemon juice, lemon zest and oregano to create the dressing. Set aside.

2.   Combine the millet, cucumber, chickpeas, spinach and parsley in a large bowl. Pour dressing over the millet mixture and toss well to coat.

3.   Garnish with black olives

Sweet Brussel Sprout Salad

Servings: 2

Total Time: 55 minutes

Ingredients

- ½ pound brussel sprouts, washed, trimmed, and halved
- 1 shallot, diced
- 1 teaspoon Himalayan salt
- ½ cup vegetable broth
- 2 tablespoons olive oil
- 1 lemon, zested
- 1 pear, cored and diced
- 1 cup almonds, toasted and chopped
- 1 teaspoon dried thyme
- ¼ teaspoon cinnamon
- 1 cup quinoa, cooked

Directions

1. Preheat the oven to 350°F/180°C.

2.   Place brussel sprouts in a deep baking dish and add in shallot and salt. Pour in vegetable broth and drizzle with olive oil.

3.   Bake the brussel sprouts for 30 minutes before adding in the lemon zest, pear, almonds, thyme and cinnamon. Toss well to combine and bake for another 15 minutes.

4.   In a large bowl, combine the quinoa and brussel sprout mixture and serve immediately.

Cherry & Fennel Salad

Servings: 2

Total Time: 10 minutes

Ingredients

- 1 cup quinoa, cooked
- 1 cup dark red cherries, pitted and halved
- 1 cup spinach, chopped
- ½ bulb fennel, thinly sliced
- ¼ cup almonds, toasted and crushed
- 1 teaspoon Himalayan salt
- 1 teaspoon black pepper, crushed
- 2 tablespoons olive oil
- 2 tablespoons apple cider vinegar
- 1 garlic clove, minced

Directions

1. In a large bowl, combine the quinoa, cherries, spinach, fennel and almonds.

2.   Whisk together the salt, pepper, olive oil, vinegar and garlic in a small bowl.

3.   Pour olive oil mixture over the quinoa and toss to coat. Serve immediately.

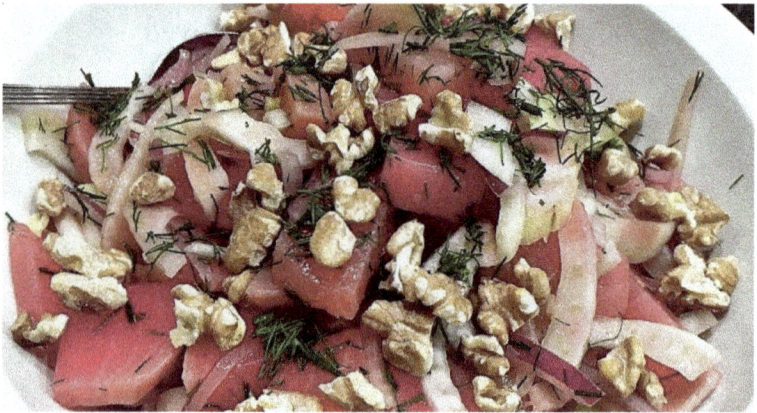

Brussel Sprouts Bowl

Servings: 2

Total Time: 35 minutes

Ingredients

- 1 bunch brussel sprouts, halved
- 1 small red onion, sliced thinly into half-moon shapes
- 2 tablespoons ghee, melted
- 1 cup brown rice, cooked
- ½ cup walnuts, chopped
- 2 tablespoons raisins
- 2 tablespoons pomegranate seeds
- 1 teaspoon Himalayan salt
- 1 teaspoon black pepper
- 1 tablespoon parsley, chopped

Directions

1. Preheat oven to 400°F/205°C. On a baking tray, place brussel sprouts and red onion. Drizzle with ghee and roast in the oven for 30 minutes or until brussel sprouts are crispy.

2.   Place brussel sprouts, brown rice, walnuts, raisins and pomegranate seeds in a large bowl. Season with salt and pepper.

3.   Garnish with parsley and serve warm.

Spicy Mexican Salad

Servings: 2

Total Time: 15 minutes

Ingredients

- 1 teaspoon coconut oil
- 1 red onion, chopped
- 1 green bell pepper, diced
- 2 garlic cloves, minced
- 1 cup quinoa, cooked
- ¼ teaspoon cayenne pepper
- ¼ teaspoon chili powder
- ⅛ teaspoon red chili flakes
- 1 teaspoon cumin
- 1 teaspoon Himalayan salt
- 1 teaspoon black pepper, crushed
- 1 15 ounce cans black beans, rinsed and drained
- 2 teaspoons lime juice
- ½ cup chopped fresh cilantro
- 1 avocado, sliced

Directions

1.   In a medium skillet over medium heat, add the oil, red onion and green bell pepper. Cook 5 minutes or until the onion and pepper are soft. Add the garlic and cook another 2 minutes.

2.   Place quinoa, cayenne pepper, chili powder, chili flakes, cumin, salt and pepper in the pan and stir well. Cook 3 minutes before adding the black beans.

3.   Continue to cook black bean and quinoa mixture for 5 minutes. Turn the heat off and stir in the lime juice and cilantro.

4.   Transfer to serving bowls and garnish with avocado slices.

Chilled Avocado Soup with Salmon

Servings: 2

Total Time: 10 minutes

Ingredients

- 3 ripe avocados, pitted and flesh removed
- 1 small shallot, chopped
- 1 tablespoon green onion, sliced
- 4 tablespoons lemon juice, divided
- 2 tablespoons full fat coconut cream
- 1 ½ cups vegetable broth
- ¼ teaspoon cumin
- ¼ teaspoon Himalayan salt
- 1 can salmon, drained and flaked
- 1 teaspoon olive oil
- 1 teaspoon black pepper, crushed
- 2 tablespoons cilantro, divided

Directions

1.	In a blender combine the avocado, shallot, green onion, 2 tablespoons of lemon juice, coconut cream, vegetable broth, cumin and salt. Let chill for at least 1 hour.

2.	In a small bowl, combine the salmon, olive oil, black pepper, 2 tablespoons lemon juice and 1 tablespoon cilantro.

3.	Place chilled avocado soup in bowls and top each with salmon, remaining cilantro. Serve immediately.

Asian Pumpkin Salad

Servings: 2

Total Time: 40 minutes

Ingredients

- 1 tablespoon white sesame seeds
- 1 tablespoon black sesame seeds
- ¼ teaspoon ground cloves
- ¼ teaspoon ground garlic
- ¼ teaspoon ground mustard
- ¼ teaspoon red chili flakes
- ½ teaspoon Himalayan salt, divided
- 2 cups pumpkin, cubed
- 1 ½ tablespoons olive oil
- 4 cups kale, stems removed and sliced into thin ribbons
- 1 tablespoon lemon juice
- ¼ cup pomegranate seeds
- ½ avocado, diced

Directions

1.   Preheat oven to 400°F/205°C. Line a baking tray with parchment paper.

2.   On a large plate, combine the white and black sesame seeds, cloves, garlic, mustard, chili flakes and half the salt.

3.   Drizzle pumpkin with 1 tablespoon olive oil and then roll each cube into the sesame seed mixture, pressing slightly to coat. Place pumpkin cubes on the parchment paper and bake for 30 minutes, turning once.

4.   While pumpkin cooks, add kale to a large bowl and drizzle with remaining olive oil, lemon juice and remaining salt. Massage gently for 3 minutes and set aside.

5.   When pumpkin is done, place on top of the kale and garnish with pomegranate seeds and avocado.

Squash & Sprouts Salad

Servings: 2

Total Time: 55 minutes

Ingredients

- 1 small butternut squash, cubed
- 2 small apples, cored and chopped
- 2 shallots, sliced
- 1 cup brussel sprouts, halved
- 2 tablespoons avocado oil
- ¼ teaspoon cinnamon
- ⅛ teaspoon turmeric
- 1 teaspoon Himalayan salt
- 1 teaspoon black pepper, crushed
- 1 tablespoon walnuts, toasted and chopped
- 1 tablespoon parsley, chopped

Directions

1. Preheat oven to 400°F/205°C. Line a baking tray with parchment paper.

2.   In a large bowl, combine the butternut squash, apples, shallots, brussel sprouts, avocado oil, cinnamon, turmeric, salt and pepper. Spread on baking tray in a single layer.

3.   Roast in the oven for 45 minutes or until vegetables are tender, tossing halfway through.

4.   Remove from oven and transfer to serving platter.

5.   Sprinkle with walnuts and parsley before serving.

Fennel Citrus Salad

Servings: 2

Total Time: 10 minutes

Ingredients

- 1 small orange, segmented
- ½ small red grapefruit, segmented
- 2 small fennel bulbs, thinly sliced
- 1 tablespoon mint, chopped
- ½ cup parsley, chopped
- 2 tablespoons fresh lemon juice
- 2 tablespoons fresh orange juice
- ¼ cup olive oil
- ⅛ teaspoon sea salt
- ½ teaspoon freshly ground black pepper
- 2 tablespoons pomegranate seeds
- ½ avocado, diced

Directions

1.   In a large bowl, combine the orange segments, grapefruit segments, fennel slices, mint and parsley.

2.   Whisk together lemon juice, orange juice, olive oil, salt and pepper. Pour over the citrus and fennel mixture. Toss well to coat.

3.   Transfer to plate and garnish with pomegranate seeds and avocado. Serve immediately.

Mushroom Wraps

Servings: 2

Total Time: 10 minutes

Ingredients

- 1 cup shiitake mushrooms, sliced

- 1 cup cremini mushrooms, sliced

- ½ cup zucchini, shredded

- ¼ cup coconut aminos

- 2 tablespoons tamari

- 3 garlic cloves, minced

- 1 tablespoon sesame oil

- ¼ teaspoon red chili flakes

- 4 Boston lettuce leaves

- 1 carrot, shredded

- 1 tablespoon cilantro

- 1 tablespoon cashews, crushed

Sauce

- ¼ cup raw coconut aminos

- 1 tablespoon raw honey

- ¼ teaspoon hot chili oil

- 1 teaspoon sesame oil

- 1 teaspoon red chili flakes

- ¼ teaspoon Himalayan salt

Directions

1.   In a large bowl, combine both mushrooms, zucchini, coconut aminos, tamari, garlic, sesame oil and chili flakes. Let sit while you prepare the Sauce.

2.   To prepare the Sauce, whisk together the Sauce ingredients in a small bowl.

3.   Assemble wraps by placing some of the mushroom mixture in a lettuce leaf and top with some carrot, cilantro and cashews. Drizzle sauce on top. Repeat with remaining ingredients and serve.

Sweet Potato Wraps

Servings: 2

Total Time: 25 minutes

Ingredients

- 4 collard greens

- ½ cup quinoa, cooked

- 1 cup spinach

- ½ red onion, thinly sliced

- 1 cup alfalfa sprouts

- 1 avocado

Sweet Potato Hummus

- 1 large sweet potato, peeled and cubed

- 1/3 cup of tahini

- ¼ cup of olive oil

- ½ lemon, juiced

- 1 garlic clove, minced

- ¼ teaspoon chili powder

- ⅛ teaspoon cinnamon powder

- ¼ teaspoon Himalayan salt

- ¼ teaspoon black pepper, crushed

Directions

1.   Place sweet potatoes in a medium saucepan and cover with water. Bring to a boil over medium-high heat and then reduce heat to a simmer and cook 15 minutes or until potatoes are tender.

2.   Drain water from the sweet potatoes and place sweet potatoes in a food processor along with the tahini, olive oil, lemon juice, garlic, chili powder, cinnamon, salt and pepper. Process until smooth.

3.   Lay out each of the collard greens before you and spread each with the Sweet Potato Hummus. Top with quinoa, spinach, onion, sprouts and avocado. Roll up and secure with toothpicks if necessary. Repeat with remaining collard greens and filling.

Refresh Green Grape Salad

Servings: 2

Total Time: 5 minutes

Ingredients

- 1 cup arugula
- 1 cup watercress
- 1 beet, shredded
- 1 cup red cabbage, shredded or chopped
- ½ avocado, diced
- 10 green grapes, halved or whole
- ½ cup walnuts, crushed
- 2 tablespoons olive oil
- ½ lemon, juiced
- ½ teaspoon Himalayan salt
- ½ teaspoon black pepper, crushed

Directions

1. Place the arugula, watercress, beet, cabbage, avocado, grapes and walnuts in a large bowl.

2.   Drizzle with olive oil, lemon juice, salt and pepper. Toss well to coat and serve immediately.

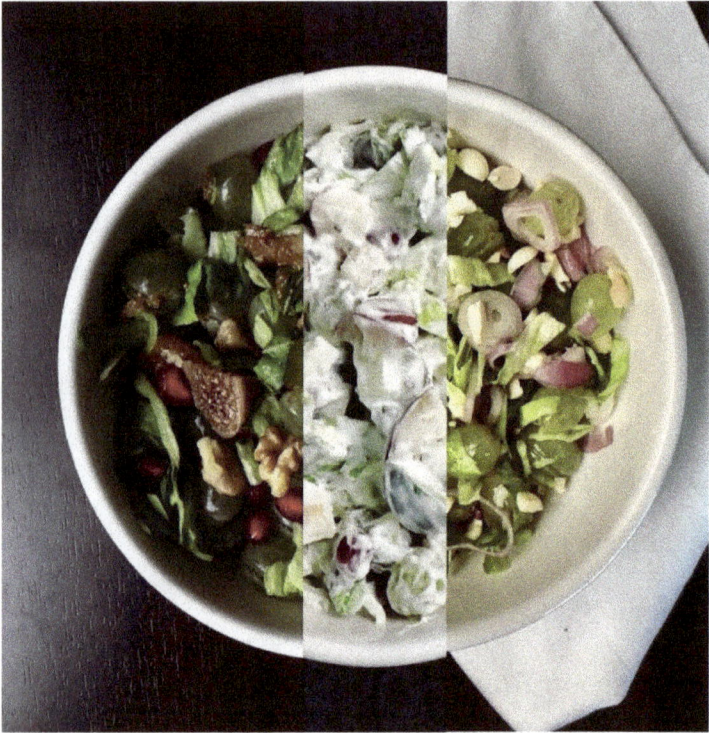

Fall Lentil Salad

Servings: 2

Total Time: 25 minutes

Ingredients

- 1 small delicata squash, sliced into ½ inch thick slices
- 2 tablespoons olive oil
- 2 teaspoons thyme leaves, chopped
- 1 garlic clove, minced
- 1 tablespoon apple cider vinegar
- 1 tablespoon lemon juice
- ½ tablespoon maple syrup
- ½ teaspoon Himalayan salt
- ½ teaspoon black pepper, crushed
- ½ cup lentils, cooked
- 2 cups spinach, stems removed and thinly sliced
- 2 tablespoons pine nuts, toasted

Directions

1.   Preheat oven to 400°F/205°C. Line a baking tray with parchment paper. In a small bowl, combine the squash, 1 tablespoon olive oil, thyme and garlic. Move the squash to the baking tray and bake in the oven for 20 minutes, flipping once halfway through.

2.   Whisk together the remaining tablespoon olive oil, apple cider vinegar, lemon juice, maple syrup, salt and pepper.

3.   In a large bowl combine the lentils, spinach, baked squash and pine nuts. Drizzle with olive oil mixture, toss to coat and serve immediately.

Brown Rice & Sprouts Salad

Servings: 2

Total Time: 5 minutes

Ingredients

- 1 cup brown rice, cooked
- 1 ½ cups of quinoa, cooked
- ½ yellow bell pepper, diced
- 5 cherry tomatoes, halved
- 2 tablespoons cilantro, chopped
- 2 tablespoons parsley, chopped
- 1 cup alfalfa sprouts
- 2 tablespoons almonds, toasted
- 1 tablespoon raisins

Dressing

- 3 tablespoons olive oil
- 1 tablespoon apple cider vinegar
- 1 tablespoon lemon juice
- 1 teaspoon maple syrup
- 1 garlic clove, minced

Directions

1.   In a large serving bowl, place brown rice and top with quinoa, yellow pepper, tomatoes, cilantro, parsley, sprouts, almonds and raisins.

2.   Whisk together Dressing ingredients in a small bowl and pour over the salad.

3.   Toss before serving.

Chopped Beet & Quinoa Salad

Servings: 2

Total Time: 40 minutes

Ingredients

- 2 medium beets, ends cut and halved

- 1 cup quinoa, cooked

- 1 stalk celery, diced small

- ½ head red cabbage, shredded

- 1 garlic clove, minced

- 1 tablespoon apple cider vinegar

- 2 tablespoons olive oil

- ½ teaspoon Himalayan salt

- ¼ teaspoon black pepper, crushed

- ¼ cup fresh mint, chopped

- ¼ cup parsley, chopped

Directions

1. Fill a medium saucepan (fitted with a steamer basket) with water until it reaches halfway. Bring water to a boil over medium

heat and then add beets to the steamer basket. Cover with a lid and reduce heat to low and cook for 30 minutes or until beets are tender.

2.   Remove beet skins by placing in a towel and rubbing off the skins. Chop the cooked beets into a small dice.

3.   In a large bowl, combine quinoa, beets, celery, cabbage, garlic, vinegar, olive oil, salt, pepper, mint and parsley. Combine well and serve immediately.

Sweet Quinoa Salad

Servings: 2

Total Time: 5 minutes

Ingredients

- 3 cups spinach, chopped
- 1 cup quinoa, cooked
- 1 shallot, thinly sliced
- 2 apples, diced
- 2 tablespoons raisins
- 2 tablespoons walnuts, toasted and crushed
- 1 handful sprouts
- 2 tablespoons avocado oil
- ½ lemon, juiced
- ½ teaspoon Himalayan salt
- ⅛ teaspoon cinnamon
- ¼ teaspoon black pepper, ground

Directions

1.   Combine spinach, quinoa, shallot, apples, raisins, walnuts and sprouts in a large bowl.

2.   Drizzle with avocado oil and pour in lemon juice. Add salt, cinnamon and black pepper.

3.   Toss well to combine and serve immediately.

Warm Spinach Salad

Servings: 2

Total Time: 15 minutes

Ingredients

- 1 tablespoon coconut oil
- ½ cup red onion, sliced thinly
- 1 garlic clove, minced
- 5 cherry tomatoes, halved
- 6 cups baby spinach
- ½ teaspoon grated lemon peel
- ½ teaspoon Himalayan salt
- ½ teaspoon black pepper
- ¼ teaspoon cinnamon
- 1 cup brown rice, cooked
- 1 tablespoon pine nuts, toasted

Directions

1.   In a medium skillet over medium heat, melt coconut oil and add onion. Cook 5 minutes and then add the garlic, cooking for an additional 1 minute.

2.   Add in tomatoes and spinach. Season with lemon peel, salt, pepper and cinnamon. Cook for 5 minutes or until spinach is wilted.

3.   Place brown rice in a bowl and top with the spinach and tomato mixture.

4.   Garnish with pine nuts and serve.

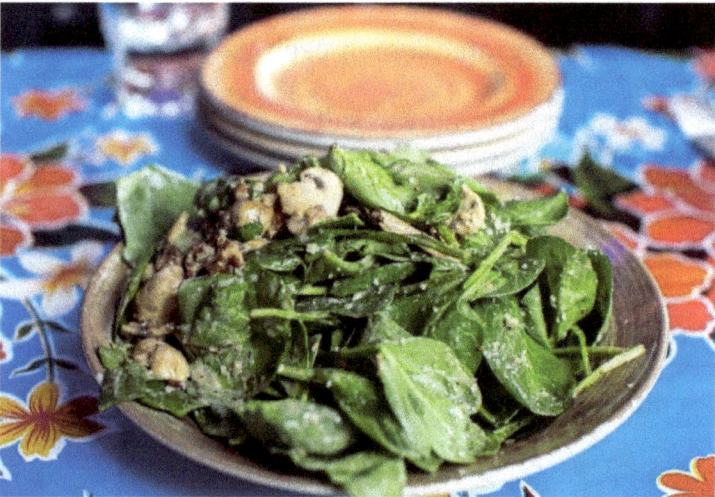

Veggie Ramen

Servings: 1

Total Time: 15 minutes

Ingredients

- 1 tablespoon of miso paste
- 1 inch ginger piece, minced
- 1 tablespoon tamari
- ½ lime, juiced
- ½ bell pepper, thinly sliced
- ¼ head of broccoli, cut into small florets
- 1 carrot, spiralized into noodles
- 4 mushrooms, stems removed and sliced
- ½ cup spinach
- ½ zucchini, spiralized
- 3 cups boiling water
- 1 tablespoon cilantro

Directions

1.   In a large bowl that has a lid, add the miso, ginger, tamari, lime juice, bell pepper, broccoli, carrot, mushrooms, spinach and zucchini.

2.   Pour boiling water into the pot, stir well a few times and then place the lid on top.

3.   Let sit 5 minutes and then garnish with cilantro and serve.

Spicy Ginger Salad

Servings: 2

Total Time: 10 minutes

Ingredients

- 3 cups kale
- 1 cup tomatoes, finely diced
- 1 tablespoon parsley, finely chopped
- 1 tablespoon raw sesame seeds
- 1 tablespoon raw pumpkin seeds
- 1 tablespoon almonds
- 1 garlic clove, minced
- ¼ teaspoon lemon zest
- ¼ teaspoon ginger, grated
- ⅛ teaspoon red chili flakes

Dressing

- 3 tablespoons olive oil
- 1 tablespoon lemon juice
- 1 tablespoon apple cider vinegar
- ¼ teaspoon fresh ginger juice

- ½ teaspoon Himalayan salt

- ¼ teaspoon cayenne pepper

- ¼ teaspoon black pepper, crushed

Directions

1.   Make the Dressing by combining the Dressing ingredients in a small bowl until well combined.

2.   In a large bowl, combine the kale, tomatoes, parsley, sesame seeds, pumpkin seeds, almonds, garlic, lemon zest, ginger and chili flakes.

3.   Pour Dressing over the kale and tomato mixture. Let rest 5 minutes before serving.

Curry Squash Soup

Servings: 2

Total Time: 25 minutes

Ingredients

- 1 tablespoon olive oil

- 1 shallot, sliced

- 1 yellow squash, diced

- ½ cup broccoli, cut into florets

- 1 teaspoon ginger, grated

- ½ teaspoon Himalayan salt

- ½ teaspoon black pepper, crushed

- ½ teaspoon cumin

- ½ teaspoon coriander

- ½ teaspoon cardamom

- ½ teaspoon turmeric

- ¼ teaspoon cinnamon

- 1 ½ cups vegetable broth

- ½ cup water

- 1 lemon, juiced

- 1 tablespoon cilantro, chopped

- 1 teaspoon pepitas, toasted

Directions

1.   Heat oil in a medium-sized pot over medium heat. Add shallot, squash, broccoli, ginger, salt, pepper, cumin, coriander, cardamom, turmeric and cinnamon.

2.   Sauté 10 minutes until vegetables are softened and then add the broth, water and lemon juice. Let come to a low boil and then reduce heat to low and simmer 10 minutes.

3.   Let cool 5 minutes and then transfer to a food processor or blender and blend until smooth.

4.   Top with cilantro and pepitas to serve.

Sweet Potato Nacho Boat

Servings: 2

Total Time: 35 minutes

Ingredients

- 2 sweet potatoes
- ½ tablespoon balsamic vinegar
- ½ teaspoon coconut aminos
- ½ tablespoon apple cider vinegar
- ½ teaspoon cayenne pepper
- ¾ cup tempeh, diced
- 1 cup spinach
- 4 black olives, sliced
- 1 tomato, diced
- 1 shallot, diced
- ½ avocado, diced

Cheese Sauce

- ¼ head of cauliflower, steamed
- ½ cup nutritional yeast
- ½ cup vegetable broth

- 1 garlic clove, minced

- ¼ teaspoon cayenne pepper

- 1 tablespoon white miso

- 1 tablespoon lemon juice

- 1 teaspoon tahini

- ½ teaspoon chili powder

Directions

1. Preheat oven to 400°F/205°C. Line a baking tray with parchment paper. Pierce sweet potatoes with a fork a few times and place on tray. Bake in the oven for 30 minutes.

2. Prepare Cheese Sauce by placing Cheese Sauce ingredients in a food processor or blender and mixing until smooth. Set aside.

3. In a small skillet over medium heat, add balsamic vinegar, coconut aminos, apple cider vinegar and cayenne. Let heat for 3 minutes and then add tempeh, tossing to coat. Cook 5 minutes until tempeh is warm and sauce is slightly reduced.

4. Cut open each sweet potato and add spinach, tempeh, olives, tomato, shallot and avocado. Drizzle cheese sauce on top and serve immediately.

Confetti Cauliflower Rice

Servings: 2

Total Time: 20 minutes

Ingredients

- ½ cauliflower head, cut into florets
- 2 teaspoons olive oil
- 2 tablespoons red onion, chopped
- ¼ cup red bell pepper, chopped
- ¼ cup green bell pepper, chopped
- 1 garlic clove, minced
- 3 tablespoons water
- 1 teaspoon chili powder
- ¼ teaspoon ground cumin
- ½ teaspoon Himalayan salt
- ½ cup black beans
- ¼ cup cilantro, chopped
- 2 tablespoons green onions, thinly sliced

Directions

1. Make cauliflower rice by processing the cauliflower florets in the food processor until it becomes a rice-like consistency.

2. Heat olive oil in a medium skillet over medium-low heat. Add onion, red bell pepper, green bell pepper and garlic. Cook for 5 minutes before adding the cauliflower rice, water, chili powder, cumin and salt.

3. Continue cooking another 5 minutes or until liquid is absorbed. Stir in black beans and cilantro and cook 2 minutes until warmed.

4. Garnish with green onions and serve.

Creamy Sweet Salad

Servings: 2

Total Time: 20 minutes

Ingredients

- ½ teaspoon coriander powder

- ¼ teaspoon cumin

- ¼ teaspoon turmeric

- ¼ teaspoon cinnamon

- ½ teaspoon Himalayan salt

- ½ teaspoon black pepper, crushed

- 1 cup unsweetened yogurt

- 2 tablespoons olive oil

- 2 cups steamed brown rice

- 3 cups celery, sliced into ½ inch pieces

- 1 cup red bell pepper, diced

- 1 cup pear, cored, peeled and cut into 1 inch pieces

- 2 tablespoons green onions, thinly sliced

- 2 tablespoons raisins

- 1 tablespoon almonds, slivered

- 4 cups mixed greens

Directions

1.   In a small bowl, combine the coriander, cumin, turmeric, cinnamon, salt and pepper. Add to the yogurt and olive oil to the spice mixture. Let sit for 15 minutes.

2.   Place brown rice, celery, bell pepper, pear, green onions, raisins and almonds in a medium sized bowl. Pour yogurt mixture into the bowl and mix well to combine.

3.   Serve brown rice and pear mixture over mixed greens.

Sweet Spinach Salad

Servings: 2

Total Time: 15 minutes

Ingredients

- ¾ cup carrots, shredded
- 1 tablespoon lime juice
- ½ cup unsweetened yogurt
- ½ cup apple, cored and diced into 1 inch pieces
- ¼ cup raisins
- ¼ cup walnuts, toasted and chopped
- 2 tablespoons parsley, chopped
- 4 cups spinach, chopped
- 1 teaspoon cinnamon
- 1 teaspoon nutmeg
- 1 teaspoon Himalayan salt
- 1 teaspoon black pepper, crushed

Directions

1. Combine all ingredients in a large bowl and mix well.

2. Chill for 10 minutes before serving.

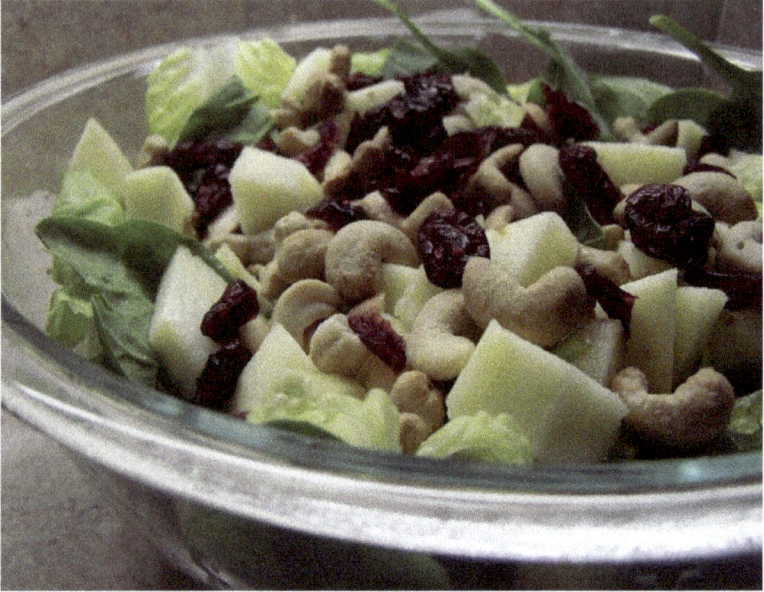

Creamy Fruit Salad

Servings: 2

Total Time: 15 minutes

Ingredients

- ¾ cup carrots, shredded
- 1 tablespoon lime juice
- ½ cup unsweetened yogurt
- ½ cup apple, cored and diced into 1 inch pieces
- ¼ cup raisins
- ¼ cup walnuts, toasted and chopped
- 2 tablespoons parsley, chopped
- 4 cups spinach, chopped
- 1 teaspoon cinnamon
- 1 teaspoon nutmeg
- 1 teaspoon Himalayan salt
- 1 teaspoon black pepper, crushed

Directions

1. Combine all ingredients in a large bowl and mix well.
2. Chill for 10 minutes before serving.

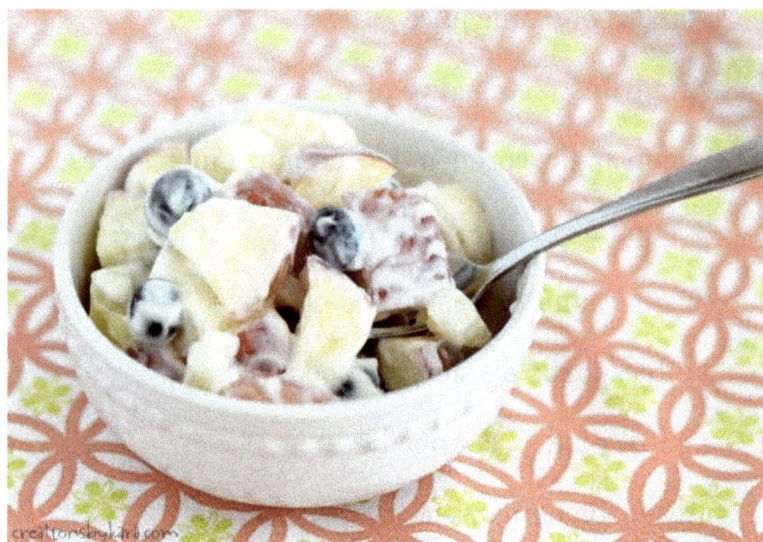

Steamed Green Bowl

Servings: 2

Total Time: 15 minutes

Ingredients

- 1 tablespoon coconut oil
- 1 medium onion, finely sliced
- 1 garlic clove, minced
- 1 teaspoon turmeric
- 1 inch piece ginger, grated
- 1 head broccoli, cut into florets
- 1 large zucchini, sliced
- ½ cup green peas
- 2 cups coconut milk
- 1 cup cashews, ground
- 2 green onions, thinly sliced
- 1 teaspoon Himalayan salt
- 2 tablespoons cilantro, chopped

Directions

1. Heat coconut oil in a medium saucepan over medium-low heat. Add onion, garlic, turmeric and ginger. Cook 5 minutes and then add broccoli, zucchini, peas and coconut milk.

2. Bring to a boil and then reduce heat to low and simmer for 15 minutes.

3. Stir in cashews, green onions, salt and cilantro and serve.

Indian Cauliflower & Potato

Servings: 2

Total Time: 35 minutes

Ingredients

- 2 tablespoons coconut oil
- 1 tablespoon ginger, grated
- 1 garlic clove, minced
- 1 medium onion, diced
- 3 tomatoes, diced
- ½ head of cauliflower, cut into florets
- ½ cup green peas
- 5 yellow potatoes, diced
- 2 teaspoons turmeric
- 1 teaspoon cumin
- 1 teaspoon coriander
- 1 teaspoon ground cardamom
- ½ teaspoon cayenne pepper
- ½ teaspoon cinnamon
- 1 teaspoon Himalayan salt

- 1 teaspoon black pepper, crushed

- 3 cups water

- 2 tablespoons green onions

Directions

1.   Heat coconut oil in a medium saucepan over medium-low heat. Add ginger, onion, garlic and tomatoes. Cook for 5 minutes and then add cauliflower, peas, potatoes, turmeric, cumin, coriander, cardamom, cayenne, cinnamon, salt and pepper.

2.   Continue cooking for 10 more minutes, stirring frequently. After 10 minutes, pour in water.

3.   Cook mixture for 20 minutes or until vegetables are soft. Toss in green onions and serve.

Berry & Vegetable Salad

Servings: 2

Total Time: 10 minutes

Ingredients

- 2 tablespoons pumpkin seeds

- 1 tablespoon almonds, crushed

- 1 carrot, shredded

- ½ red bell pepper, sliced

- 1 tablespoon parsley, chopped

- 4 leaves of kale, stems removed and sliced into thin ribbons

- 1 shallot, sliced thinly

- 1 avocado

- 1 small cucumber, diced

- 3 tablespoons olive oil

- 1 lemon, juiced

- ½ head of red cabbage, shredded

- 1 cup alfalfa sprouts

- ½ small tangerine, sliced into segments

- ½ cup raspberries

Directions

1.   Add all ingredients to a large bowl. Toss well to combine and coat the vegetables with the oil and lemon juice.

2.   Serve immediately.

Shredded Cauliflower Salad

Servings: 2

Total Time: 10 minutes

Ingredients

- ½ head of cauliflower, chopped into small pieces (like rice) in food processor
- 1 cup spinach, finely chopped
- 2-3 leaves kale, stems removed and finely chopped
- ¼ cup cilantro, finely chopped
- 2 green onions, sliced
- 1 tablespoon chives
- 1 ripe avocado, mashed
- 1 tablespoon tamari
- 1 teaspoon coconut aminos
- 1 lime, juiced
- ½ teaspoon red chili flakes
- 2 tablespoons cashews, toasted and crushed
- 2 tablespoons pumpkin seeds, toasted and crushed
- 1 tablespoon flaxseeds

- 1 teaspoon cayenne pepper

- 1 teaspoon cumin

- ½ teaspoon Himalayan salt

- 2 teaspoons coconut oil, melted

- 1 teaspoon raw honey

Directions

1. In a large bowl, add cauliflower, spinach, kale, cilantro, green onions and chives.

2. Whisk together mashed avocado, tamari, coconut aminos, lime juice and chili flakes until smooth. Pour over the salad and massage gently.

3. In a small bowl, combine cashews, pumpkin seeds, flaxseeds, cayenne pepper, cumin, salt, coconut oil and honey together.

4. Top salad with the nut/seed mixture.

Root Vegetable & Citrus Bowl

Servings: 2

Total Time: 50 minutes

Ingredients

- ¼ cup orange juice
- ¼ cup grapefruit juice
- 1 teaspoon Dijon mustard
- 1 tablespoon apple cider vinegar
- 1 teaspoon coconut oil
- ½ teaspoon sea salt
- ½ teaspoon black pepper, crushed
- ¼ teaspoon cayenne pepper
- ½ red onion, quartered
- 1 sweet potato, cut into chunks
- 1 carrot, cut into chunks
- 1 small beet, peeled and cut into large chunks
- 2 garlic cloves, peeled and left whole
- ½ inch piece ginger, grated
- ¼ cup parsley, chopped

- 2 tablespoons rosemary

- 1 ½ cups quinoa, cooked

- 2 tablespoons parsley (for garnishing)

- 2 tablespoons pumpkin seeds

Directions

1. Preheat oven to 400°F/205°C.

2. Whisk together the orange juice, grapefruit juice, mustard, vinegar, coconut oil, salt, pepper and cayenne in a small bowl.

3. In a large bowl combine the onion, potato, carrot, beet, garlic, ginger, parsley, rosemary. Pour citrus juice mixture over the vegetables and toss to coat.

4. Place vegetables on a parchment lined baking tray and place in the oven for 45 minutes, turning once.

5. Remove vegetables and place on top of quinoa. Garnish with parsley and pumpkin seeds and serve.

Veggie Jambalaya

Servings: 2

Total Time: 5 minutes plus 6 hours slow cooker time

Ingredients

- ½ eggplant, peeled and cut into ½ inch pieces
- 1 small zucchini, cut into ½ inch pieces
- 1 small yellow squash, cut into ½ inch pieces
- 1 celery stalk, diced
- ¼ cup olive oil
- ½ yellow onion, finely diced
- 1 garlic clove, minced
- 1 jalapeño, seeds removed and finely diced
- ½ red bell pepper, diced
- 2 small tomatoes, diced
- ⅛ teaspoon cayenne pepper
- ¼ teaspoon smoked paprika
- 1 teaspoon thyme
- 1 tablespoon apple cider vinegar
- 1 teaspoon Himalayan salt

- 1 teaspoon black pepper, crushed

- 2 cups water

- ½ uncooked brown rice

- 2 tablespoons green onions, sliced

Directions

1. In a slow cooker, add all ingredients except the rice and green onions. Stir to combine and place lid on the slow cooker.

2. Cook on low for 5 hours.

3. After 5 hours, stir in the rice and ensure there is enough water to cover entire mixture. Cook another 40 minutes on low or until rice is tender.

4. Transfer to bowls and garnish with green onions.

Detox Salad

Servings: 2

Total Time: 10 minutes

Ingredients

- 3 beets, peeled, roasted and diced

- 3 green onions, sliced

- 1 lime, juiced

- ¼ cup raisins

- 3 cups watercress

- 1 pear, diced

- 1 celery stalk, diced

- ½ avocado, diced

- ½ cup almonds, toasted and crushed

Dressing

- 1 garlic clove, minced

- ¼ teaspoon Himalayan salt

- 1 teaspoon coriander

- 1 teaspoon cumin

- ½ teaspoon cinnamon

- ½ teaspoon turmeric

- ½ teaspoon fresh ginger, grated

- 1 lemon, juiced

- 6 tablespoons of avocado oil

Directions

1.   In a large bowl, combine beets, green onions, lime juice, raisins, watercress, pear, celery, avocado and almonds. Toss well to combine.

2.   In a small bowl or jar, combine all the Dressing ingredients together. Whisk well to combine.

3.   Pour Dressing over the beet and watercress mixture and toss well to coat.

4.   Serve immediately.

Alkaline Falafel Salad

Servings: 2

Total Time: 35 minutes

Ingredients

- 2 cups kale, stems removed and thinly sliced
- 1 cup radicchio, sliced
- ½ cucumber, diced
- ½ tomato, diced
- 1 lemon, juiced
- 2 tablespoons olive oil
- 1 teaspoon Himalayan salt
- 1 teaspoon black pepper crushed
- ¼ cup pomegranate seeds
- 1 avocado, diced
- ¼ cup parsley, chopped

Falafels

- 1 teaspoon olive oil
- ½ red onion, diced
- 1 garlic clove, minced

- ½ cup brown lentils, cooked

- ¼ cup chickpeas

- ¼ cup peas, cooked

- ¼ cup parsley, chopped

- ¼ cup tablespoons tahini

- ¼ teaspoon cumin

- 1 teaspoon Himalayan salt

Directions

1. Preheat oven to 375°F/190°C.

2. Make the Falafels by heating a teaspoon of olive oil in a medium skillet over medium heat. Add the onion and garlic and cook 5 minutes until soft. Add to a food processor along with the lentils, chickpeas, peas and parsley. Pulse until mixture starts to come together, then add the tahini, cumin and salt.

3. Form Falafels by forming into balls using 1 ½ tablespoons of the mixture and placing on a baking tray lined with parchment paper. Bake the Falafels for 15-20 minutes.

4. In a large bowl, combine the kale, radicchio, cucumber, tomato, lemon juice, olive oil, salt and pepper. Toss to coat well.

5. Place Falafels, pomegranate seeds, avocado and parsley on top of the salad and serve immediately.

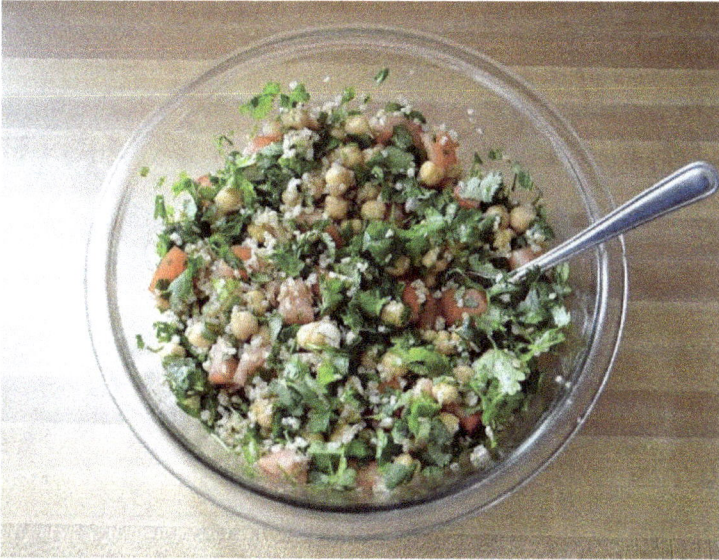

Chopped Salad

Servings: 2

Total Time: 10 minutes

Ingredients

- ½ head romaine lettuce
- 1 cucumber, diced
- 1 tomato, diced
- ½ green bell pepper, diced
- ¼ cup green onions, diced
- ¼ cup black olives, chopped
- 2 tablespoons red onion, diced
- 2 tablespoons parsley, chopped

Dressing

- 1 tablespoon lemon juice
- 2 tablespoons apple cider vinegar
- 1 garlic clove, minced
- ¼ teaspoon Himalayan salt
- ⅛ teaspoon pepper
- ½ teaspoon dried oregano

- 1/3 cup olive oil

Directions

1.   Make Dressing by whisking together all the Dressing ingredients together.

2.   Place the lettuce, cucumber, tomato, bell pepper, green onions, olives, red onion and parsley in a large bowl. Drizzle with Dressing and toss to coat.

Carrot & Quinoa Bowl

Servings: 2

Total Time: 30 minutes

Ingredients

- 1 cup warm water
- 1 tablespoon miso
- 1 tablespoon olive oil
- 1 bunch carrots, scrubbed and cut into large chunks
- 1 fennel bulb, thinly sliced
- 2 cups quinoa, cooked
- ½ lemon, juiced
- 3 tablespoons parsley, chopped
- ¼ teaspoon Himalayan salt
- 2 tablespoons black sesame seeds
- 2 tablespoons green onions, sliced

Directions

1. Whisk together water and miso in a small bowl

2.   Heat olive oil in a large skillet over medium heat. Add carrots and fennel bulb in a single layer and cook 3 minutes before flipping. Continue to cook for another 3 minutes.

3.   Pour miso and water mixture into the pan and reduce heat to low. Cook, with the lid on, for 20 minutes.

4.   While carrots are cooking, combine the quinoa, lemon juice, parsley and salt in a medium bowl.

5.   Place cooked carrot and fennel mixture over the quinoa, sprinkle with the sesame seeds, green onions and serve.

Seaweed & Carrot Rollups

Servings: 2

Total Time: 35 minutes

Ingredients

- ¼ ounce dried wakame

- 1 carrot, spiralized

- 8 ounces extra-firm tofu, drained and cut into 2 long rectangles

- ½ avocado, pitted, peeled and thinly sliced

- 2 sprouted tortillas or large lettuce leaves (such as Bibb lettuce)

- 1 tablespoon sesame seeds

- 1 tablespoon green onion, sliced

Dressing

- 1 teaspoon reduced-sodium tamari

- 1 teaspoon coconut aminos

- 1 teaspoon toasted sesame oil

- ¼ teaspoon red chili flakes

Directions

1.   In a large bowl, place wakame and cover with cold water. Let sit for 10 minutes and then drain and dry.

2.   In a small bowl, stir together the tamari, coconut aminos, sesame oil and red chili flakes to form the Dressing.

3.   Place half the wakame, carrot, tofu and avocado in one of the wraps or lettuce leaves. Drizzle the Dressing on top and sprinkle with sesame seeds and green onion.

4.   Repeat with the remaining ingredients and roll up each one. Secure with a toothpick and serve.

Middle Eastern Salad

Servings: 2

Total Time: 15 minutes

Ingredients

- 4 small eggplants, sliced into ⅛ inch thick rounds
- 1 teaspoon Himalayan salt
- 1 tablespoon olive oil
- ½ cup lentils, cooked
- ½ cup parsley, chopped
- ½ cup dill, chopped
- ¼ cup walnuts, toasted
- ¼ cup raisins
- 1 ½ cups arugula
- 1 ½ cups spinach
- 1 lemon, zested and juiced
- 3 tablespoons olive oil
- ½ teaspoon Himalayan salt
- ½ teaspoon black pepper, crushed

Spice Blend

- ¼ cup sesame seeds, toasted

- 2 tablespoons dried thyme

- 1 tablespoon dried marjoram

- 1 tablespoon dried oregano

- ½ teaspoon Himalayan salt

Directions

1.   Place eggplant rounds on a paper towel and sprinkle with the teaspoon of salt. Allow to rest while continuing with the other directions.

2.   While eggplant rests, prepare Spice Blend by combining all the Spice Blend ingredients in a small bowl and mixing well.

3.   Brush eggplant with olive oil on both sides and sprinkle with Spice Blend. Place in a grill pan that has been preheated over medium-high heat. Cook for 5 minutes on each side or until tender.

4.   In a small bowl, combine the lentils, parsley, dill, walnuts and raisins. Place on top of the arugula and spinach that has been combined in a large serving bowl. Squeeze lemon juice and drizzle olive oil on top and season with salt and pepper. Toss well to combine.

5.   Place eggplant slices on top of the greens and lentil mixture and serve.

Tropical Tofu Salad

Servings: 2

Total Time: 10 minutes

Ingredients

- ½ mango, diced
- ½ cup pineapple, diced
- 1 carrot, shredded
- ½ red bell pepper, thinly sliced
- 7 ounces firm tofu, drained and diced
- ¼ cup cilantro, chopped
- 1 cup arugula
- ¼ cup sesame seeds, toasted
- 2 tablespoons green onions

Dressing

- 1 tablespoon white miso paste
- 2 teaspoons warm water
- 2 teaspoons coconut aminos
- 1 lime, juiced
- ¼ teaspoon cayenne pepper

Directions

1.   Make Dressing by combining the Dressing ingredients in a small bowl and whisking well. If mixture is too thick or miso won't dissolve, add more warm water.

2.   In a large bowl, combine the mango, pineapple, carrot, bell pepper, tofu, cilantro and arugula together.

3.   Drizzle Dressing on top and toss to coat.

4.   Sprinkle with sesame seeds and green onions.

Sweet Broccoli Quinoa Bowl

Servings: 2

Total Time: 10 minutes

Ingredients

- 5 tablespoons water
- 2 tablespoons tahini
- 1 teaspoon turmeric
- ½ teaspoon cinnamon
- ½ lemon, juiced
- 1 teaspoon maple syrup
- 1 head broccoli, florets finely chopped
- ¼ cup red grapes, halved
- ¼ cup almonds, chopped
- 1 cup quinoa, cooked
- 1 teaspoon Himalayan salt
- 1 teaspoon black pepper, crushed

Directions

1.   In a small bowl, whisk together the water, tahini, turmeric, cinnamon, lemon juice and maple syrup until smooth.

2.   In a large bowl, combine the broccoli, grapes, almonds and quinoa.

3.   Pour tahini sauce over the broccoli and quinoa mixture and add salt and pepper.

4.   Toss well to coat and serve.

Cooling Mint Salad

Servings: 2

Total Time: 10 minutes

Ingredients

- 2 cups spinach, chopped
- 2 cups radishes, thinly sliced
- 1 cucumber, diced
- 2 small red onions, cut in half and thinly sliced
- ¼ cup almonds, sliced

Mint & Citrus Dressing

- 1 tablespoon raw honey
- ¼ cup orange juice
- 1 tablespoon lemon juice
- 4 tablespoons olive oil
- 1 teaspoon Himalayan salt
- 1 teaspoon black pepper, crushed
- 1 cup fresh mint leaves, chopped

Directions

1. In a small bowl, whisk together the Mint & Citrus Dressing ingredients.

2. In a large bowl, combine the spinach, radishes, cucumber, red onion and almonds. Pour in Mint & Citrus Dressing and toss to coat.

3. Serve immediately.

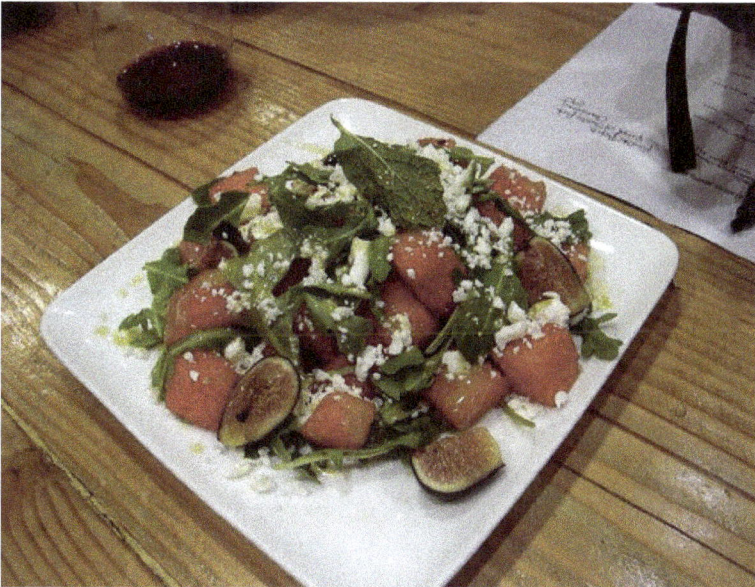

Antioxidant Salad

Servings: 2

Total Time: 10 minutes

Ingredients

- 1 tablespoon coconut oil
- 1 teaspoon apple cider vinegar
- ¾ cup almonds, toasted
- 1 garlic clove, minced
- ½ cup quinoa, cooked
- 1/3 cup raisins
- ¼ cup blueberries
- 2 cups spinach, torn
- 1 handful of sesame seeds
- 1 teaspoon Himalayan salt

Directions

1. In a large bowl, toss together all ingredients and mix well.
2. Chill 5 minutes and serve.

Minted Quinoa Salad

Servings: 2

Total Time: 5 minutes

Ingredients

- ½ cup red quinoa, cooked
- ½ red bell pepper, diced
- ½ green bell pepper, diced
- ½ cucumber, diced
- 6 ounces chickpeas, cooked
- 1/3 cup mint leaves, thinly sliced
- ½ red onion, thinly sliced
- 2 tablespoons parsley, chopped
- 1 tablespoon pine nuts, toasted

Dressing

- 3 tablespoons olive oil
- 2 tablespoons lemon juice
- 1 tablespoon lemon zest
- ½ teaspoon Himalayan salt
- 1 teaspoon oregano

Directions

1.	In a large bowl, combine quinoa, red and green bell peppers, cucumber, chickpeas, mint leaves and onion.

2.	In a small bowl, whisk together the olive oil, lemon juice, lemon zest, salt and oregano.

3.	Pour Dressing over the quinoa and vegetables.

4.	Garnish with parsley and pine nuts before serving.

Sweet & Sour Seaweed Salad

Servings: 2

Total Time: 10 minutes plus 20 minutes soaking time

Ingredients

- 3 tablespoons arame, soaked 10 minutes and then drained
- 1 tablespoon wakame, soaked 10 minutes and then drained
- 3 beets, grated
- 1 white radish, grated
- 1 shallot, sliced
- 2 cups spinach, chopped
- ½ cup mango, diced
- 2 tablespoons dried cherries, soaked 20 minutes and drained
- 2 tablespoons black sesame seeds
- ½ avocado, sliced

Dressing

- ½ cup white miso
- ¼ cup apple cider vinegar
- 1 lemon, juiced

- 3 tablespoons ginger, minced

- 1 garlic clove, minced

- ¼ cup avocado oil

- 1 tablespoon maple syrup

- Few drops of toasted sesame oil

Directions

1. In a large bowl, combine arame, wakame, beets, radish, shallot, spinach, mango and cherries.

2. In a blender, combine the Dressing ingredients until well combined.

3. Pour Dressing over the seaweed mixture, garnish with the sesame seeds and avocado and serve immediately.

Nutty Snap Pea & Quinoa Salad

Servings: 2

Total Time: 10 minutes

Ingredients

- 1 tablespoon extra-virgin olive oil
- 1 lemon, zested and juiced
- 1 tablespoon orange juice
- ⅛ teaspoon red chili flakes
- ⅛ teaspoon salt
- ⅛ teaspoon black pepper, crushed
- 1 ½ cup snap peas
- 1 cup quinoa, cooked
- ½ red onion, thinly sliced
- ¼ cup mint leaves, thinly sliced
- 1 tablespoon almonds, slivered and toasted
- 1 tablespoon pine nuts, toasted

Directions

1.   In a small bowl, whisk together the olive oil, lemon juice and zest, orange juice, red chili flakes, salt and black pepper.

2.   Combine the snap peas, quinoa, red onion and mint. Pour olive oil and citrus juice mixture over the quinoa and snap peas and toss to combine.

3.   Garnish with almonds and pine nuts before serving.

Grab & Go Green Wraps

Servings: 2

Total Time: 10 minutes

Ingredients

- 1 cup green peas, steamed
- 1 small avocado
- 1 small lime, juiced
- ¼ cup fresh cilantro leaves, chopped
- 1 shallot, diced
- ¼ - ½ jalapeño pepper, seeds removed and diced
- ¼ teaspoon Himalayan salt
- 4 large collard grccns
- ½ red bell pepper, seeds removed and thinly sliced
- 1 carrot, julienned

Directions

1.   In a food processor or blender, combine the peas, avocado, lime, cilantro, shallot, jalapeno and salt. Process until combined but still has some texture.

2.   Lay out a collard green in front of you and spread pea avocado mixture on top. Add some bell pepper and carrot strips. Roll up the collard green and secure with a toothpick.

3.   Repeat with remaining ingredients and serve.